Shaken

Shaken

Coping with Parkinson's Disease

Robert S. Magill PhD and Margaret G. Magill MS

To order additional copies of this book, contact:
Xlibris Corporation
1-888-795-4274
www.Xlibris.com
Orders@Xlibris.com
73790

We want to thank the people who have helped us cope with this illness and have made it possible for us to write this book.

Thank you! Thank you! To:

Our families: especially our children, Andrew and Joanna, our son-in-law, Aaron; and our grandchildren, Derek and Asia for their love, support, and help.

Our kind and helpful Care Manager Doreen Corso R.N.

Our caregivers: Brittany Gobbeo, C.N.A.; and Yancy Greer, C.N.A.; who have provided assistance, strength, and support on many levels including in the editing and typing of the manuscript.

Our doctors and specialists of the Regional Parkinson Center at Aurora Sinai Medical Center – Milwaukee: Jay Blankenship, M.S.W., C.F.R.E.; Trevor Hyde, Ph.D.; Jonathon Klein, B.A.; Gary Leo, D.O.; Paul Mamerow, P.A.-C.; Paul Nausieda, M.D., Medical Director; JoAnn Povlich, L.P.N.; Stacy Ory, B.A.; and Dacy Reimer, R.N., B.S.N., C.C.R.C.

Our friends and neighbors: Dr. Bruce and Dr. Betsy Axelrod, Mary Lou Ballweg and Jim Dorr, Jan Letven and Lorin Stein, and Ann Demorest.

DEDICATION

We dedicate *Shaken* to everyone learning to cope with
Parkinson's Disease and everyone who is part of a
support system for someone who has PD.
We honor their courage and persistence.

CONTENTS

Robert S. Magill, Ph.D.

Professor Emeritus

Helen Bader School of Social Welfare

The University of Wisconsin-Milwaukee

Milwaukee, WI 53211

Margaret G. Magill, MS

magill@uwm.edu

INTRODUCTION

I do not want to have Parkinson's disease (PD). Nobody does. For almost two years, I denied, repressed, and ignored the irrefutable evidence that I was showing symptoms of PD. I ignored the pleadings of my wife and friends that I go to a physician for a diagnosis of my symptoms. Early in the process, a friend, whose father had PD, told me that my posture and my walk were signs of Parkinson's disease. "A lot she knows," I said to myself. "I can tough this out without seeing a physician."

The repression and denial lasted almost two years. Finally, I agreed to consult with my internist. He examined me by moving my arms and legs. He then declared that I did not have Parkinson's disease. My doctor failed to see the evidence. It is not unusual for doctors to fail to diagnose Parkinson's disease. Precise knowledge of the illness is relatively minimal among many physicians. While there are similarities among people with Parkinson's, differences in symptoms exist as well. This fact makes diagnosis difficult for physicians not very familiar with the disease.

Despite my doctor's failure to diagnose PD, evidence continued to mount that something was seriously wrong with my body. I walked stooped over and shuffled my feet. I had what was called the Parkinson's mask. My face, usually quite expressive, was immobile. My sleep was very irregular as well. I was up often during the night because my arm and leg muscles would not relax long enough for me to remain asleep. During the day, I felt sleepy and needed frequent naps. I was stiff much of the time and had lost some of my fine motor skills. Because of problems with depth perception and spatial relationships, I experienced serious difficulties when driving a car. Still, I did not see the need for evaluation by another doctor.

Looking back, I think I was scared. I felt better without a frightening diagnosis. However, in this case, ignorance was not bliss. My deteriorating condition continued to gnaw at me.

Gradually I came to an understanding that I had an illness. Still, recognizing that one needs help is not the same as actually making a doctor's appointment. I felt that I was strong and could fight this illness on my own. Knowing that the human body has remarkable recuperative powers, I decided that my body would fight and defeat the disease, whatever it was.

However, my body did not solve the problem. My symptoms got worse, and I became increasingly difficult to live with. I only can imagine what I put my wife through.

Finally, my resistance dissipated when some very close friends, Bruce & Betsy Axelrod, convinced me to see a specialist in neurologic diseases. I chose Dr. Paul Nausieda, the neurologist who directs the Regional Parkinson Center at Aurora Sinai Medical Center in Milwaukee, Wisconsin. The center has become one of the largest Parkinson's clinics in the country. Dr. Nausieda and his team treat patients and research the causes and treatment of Parkinson's disease. During the first appointment, the doctor said that I had an immobile face, which he called the Parkinson's mask. He observed my walk and evaluated it as the slow, shuffling walk of a person with Parkinson's. He noted that I stood leaning forward and bent over. He very quickly diagnosed my symptoms as characteristic of Parkinson's disease.

Accepting this diagnosis became my official acknowledgment that my life had been changing substantially and would continue to change in many ways.

Before developing PD, I led a full and active life. Born in 1941, I grew up through the 1940s, the 1950s, and the 1960s. The 1940s and 1950s were decades of very conservative thinking and behavior. I grew up in a two-parent family typical of the two decades. My father worked long hours at his business. Keeping house and raising my disabled younger brother and me, my mother worked hard at home and was active in the community.

People did not talk a lot about their family problems. Getting outside help for coping with family problems occurred infrequently. In comparison, since the 1960s, many people have been seeking counseling.

In contrast to the 1950s, the 1960s were a time of experimentation and change. Industrialization increased, and the computer age began. These changes led the way to more medical research and more open communication within the family about problems, illness, and disabilities.

After graduating from Antioch College, I received a master's degree from the Columbia University School of Social Work. Later, I earned a Ph.D. in Social Service Administration from the University of Chicago.

Early in my career, I worked at a settlement house. While at Columbia, I was employed at an agency serving people who were visually impaired. Also, I worked at the Urban League on issues of discrimination in housing. Next, I moved to North Carolina to supervise neighborhood workers in the Poverty Program. In Pittsburg, I worked at a social planning agency. In 1969, I joined the faculty of the School of Social Welfare at the University of Wisconsin–Milwaukee.

Peggy grew up in the 1940s, the 1950s, and the 1960s as well. She and her family experienced the same changes in societal norms and attitudes, from very conservative to open to change.

After high school, Peggy left the East Coast to experience life in the Midwest at Carleton College. Four years later, she returned to the East Coast to attend the School of Social Work at Columbia University.

Upon graduation, Peggy joined me in moving to North Carolina to work in the Poverty Program. She helped low-income parents and their children with school problems and dysfunctional family interactions.

Peggy and I were married after leaving North Carolina. Despite the typical stresses and strains, we have enjoyed a wonderful marriage. We have two children, Andrew and Joanna, a grandson, Derek, and a granddaughter, Asia. We all have a strong sense of family. Still, Parkinson's disease has contributed to the difficulties and tensions. On our own and with help, we are doing a very good job of coping. Peggy remains my companion, my best friend, and now also my caregiver.

Before PD, I thrived in the academic environment of the School of Social Welfare at the University of Wisconsin–Milwaukee. I loved teaching, interacting with students, reading, and writing. I have written two academic books and many scholarly articles. I have given formal academic papers twice in China, and in England, France, Spain, the Netherlands, Sweden, and Canada. In recognition of my accomplishments and contributions to the field of social welfare, my department promoted me to full professor in 1995.

Later, at the height of my academic career, Parkinson's disease struck with great force. Three years later, I retired because fatigue, memory loss, aphasia, and depression made me too disabled to continue teaching.

Shaken—Coping with Parkinson's Disease developed from a desire to help people with Parkinson's disease think about and cope with what may lie ahead. Topics include the nature of Parkinson's disease and the effects of PD on the personality and mental health of individuals and their families. One section focuses specifically on the various feelings that develop from needing, receiving, and refusing help. Also discussed are the effects of PD on going out in public and communicating with others about PD. Another chapter explores the implications of having a chronic illness. Hopefully, some of our efforts to fight the disease and try to live productive and satisfying lives will be helpful to others struggling with Parkinson's.

Shaken presents information, ideas, and suggestions for understanding PD and living with it. Writing a book about Parkinson's disease is a challenge because people with Parkinson's are different from each other, and their symptoms may differ in types and severity. However, many common issues arise for most people with PD. For example, depression is prevalent because the lack of sufficient, naturally produced dopamine can result in a depressed mood. Further, living with the symptoms and pervasive limitations caused by Parkinson's disease can lead to and exacerbate depression.

The chapters explore emotions stemming from having a chronic illness. They include frustration, anger, fear, and sadness. Complicated emotions about loss of some independence and increase in dependence arise from needing to accept help from others. Making arrangements for assistance can trigger a variety of emotions as well. All these emotions affect the relationships among the person with PD, the significant other, and other family members. Everyone's functioning is affected. Family dynamics change.

Shaken is organized from the perspective of the person with Parkinson's and of the significant other as they interact with each other and with people from various parts of their lives. Throughout the book, the reader can see some of the effects of Parkinson's disease on the individual, on the marriage, and on the family. *Shaken* discusses what people with PD might do to live a less stressful and more satisfying life. With that goal, we focus on the person with Parkinson's as a whole person and not as just a patient. In the midst of stressful lives, this broader focus is important for maintaining a good quality of life.

CHAPTER 1

Parkinson's Disease—A Definition

Parkinson's disease is a progressive neurologic disorder caused by the death of cells that produce a chemical called dopamine. Dopamine is a neurotransmitter that sends signals from the brain that tell the body when, where, and how much to move. Dopamine also plays a major role in generating and maintaining mood. In Parkinson's disease, the deficiency of dopamine can produce various symptoms. By the time symptoms appear, as many as 80 percent of cells that produce dopamine no longer function (Parkinson's Action Network 2002, 2).

According to the Parkinson's Disease Foundation, "As many as one million Americans live with Parkinson's disease, which is more than the combined number of people diagnosed with multiple sclerosis, muscular dystrophy and Lou Gehrig's disease. An estimated seven to 10 million people worldwide are living with Parkinson's disease. Approximately 60,000 Americans are diagnosed with PD each year, and this number does not reflect the thousands of cases that go undetected. Incidence of Parkinson's increases with age, but an estimated four percent of people with PD are diagnosed before the age of 50 (PDF 2011)." "While most people tend to show symptoms by their mid 50's . . . Parkinson's affects men and women, all races and ethnic groups. It is anticipated that the incidence of Parkinson's will increase as more members of the baby boom generation enter mid-life (Parkinson's Action Network 2002)."

There is growing evidence that pollution in the environment is a contributing cause of Parkinson's disease. Most experts agree that there is probably more than one cause. Some individuals may inherit a genetic tendency to develop PD.

James Parkinson, a British physician, diagnosed the disease in 1817. Later the disease was named after him. His paper, *An Essay on the Shaking Palsy*, described the major symptoms of Parkinson's disease.

The most common symptoms of PD include tremors, muscle stiffness, poor balance, slowness of movement (bradykinesia), difficulty walking, freezing, and falling. Also common are difficulty focusing and swallowing. Some people produce extra saliva.

Tremoring usually begins in a part of the body and can expand to other parts. It is most prevalent when a person is resting or under stress. Tremoring can call unwelcome attention to the person with PD.

Rigidity, including stiffness of the limbs and sometimes of the trunk, results in postural instability, impaired balance, and inadequate coordination. People with PD often lean forward and fall easily. They have a tendency to walk with a stooped posture, with the head bowed and the shoulders dropped (Nauseida 2001).

Bradykinesia, or pronounced slowness of movement, involves the loss of the natural pace and rhythm of movement. Bradykinesia can include a hesitation in starting to move, a shuffling gait, taking small steps rather than big ones, and freezing. Bradykinesia is a particularly frustrating aspect of PD. One moment the person can move easily, and the next moment he or she may freeze. The freezing may lead to a fall.

Loss of manual dexterity and fine motor control also are symptoms of PD. The loss of fine motor control often results in illegible handwriting, difficulty using utensils, and problems with dressing.

At first, the symptoms of this progressive disease can be subtle, often almost imperceptible. As PD advances, bradykinesia can become more pronounced. Some people with PD develop involuntary and uncontrollable movements that are classified as dyskinesia. Other severe problems that may develop with advanced Parkinson's disease include problems with swallowing, falling and being unable to walk more than short distances. Some people with PD resist leaving the house. Deficits in cognition may cause for some who have PD additional substantial difficulties in coping with everyday activities. Coping with later stages of PD demands a lot of courage and persistence.

Many people compare Parkinson's disease and Alzheimer's disease. Alzheimer's attacks the mind, although the body may continue to function. "Parkinson destroys the body's ability to function. Those with very advanced PD eventually may have difficulty moving, swallowing, and speaking (ibid., 2)." Parkinson's may attack the mind as well. Some symptoms are quite similar and others quite different.

Parkinson's symptoms often can be controlled for some time by medications, such as Sinemet, which replaces some of the body's missing dopamine. Relief depends in part on discovering the most effective medication and its dosage and taking the medication regularly.

In the long term, the medication can cause side effects and can lose effectiveness. Parkinson's progression is often slower than some other neurologic diseases, such as Lou Gehrig's disease and Huntington's disease. Eventually, for most people with PD, current medication cannot compensate sufficiently for the extent of the death of dopamine-producing cells.

The inability to control one's movements affects self-esteem and one's sense of being part of the surrounding world. Limited mobility can be devastating and affects almost all aspects of life. Taken for granted by most of us, mobility is a serious problem for people with Parkinson's.

Parkinson's disease can cause significant problems with thinking. PD can interfere with the ability to create and follow a sequence. Understanding, learning, and following sequences can become a challenge because of short-term memory loss, difficulty concentrating, and confusion. Finishing a task or any activity can be difficult for the same reasons.

As a result, people with Parkinson's are not always reliable. They can forget what to buy at the grocery store. Phone messages are not always complete or are forgotten totally. Tools are left in the wrong place. The bed isn't made. Dirty clothes can end up on the floor or on a convenient chair rather than in the laundry basket.

Parkinson's disease is a disease that originates in the brain and affects both the mind and body. Etiology includes contact with pollutants in the environment. Recent studies suggest an association between pesticides and herbicides and Parkinson's disease (Marty 2002, 1; Planet Ark 2000). Some researchers feel that there is a genetically transmitted vulnerability to develop Parkinson's (Nauseida 2001). Also, some doctors think a traumatic assault to the brain may be a factor. A significant virus could be one type of traumatic assault (Hyde 2011).

Parkinson's affects all aspects of a person's life from self-concept and self-esteem to relationships with family and friends, performance at work, and involvement in leisure time activities.

CHAPTER 2

Parkinson's Disease and the Family

I am lucky to have a wonderful wife. I am sure I couldn't cope with this disease without her. She knows me well enough to help when I need help and to step back if she thinks I can solve the problem myself. She has worked hard to be supportive and understanding and to ease my way.

Peggy and I have a lot of similar interests. They have kept our marriage fresh. While I was sufficiently mobile, we regularly hiked in the woods and canoed with our dog. We loved to read, see films and plays, and enjoy art. Travelling gave us lots of pleasure. Biking provided exercise and fun. Getting together with friends was important to our life together.

Now we still enjoy being with our friends and walking our dog. We continued to read, go to films and plays and discuss them. As before, we love going to art museums, galleries, and fairs. Still, with Parkinson's disease ever present, less time and energy are available for all of these activities. We must adjust to the loss of some activities. These losses bring sadness. In addition to these losses, there are disagreements, as in any marriage. We have experienced stressful periods as we adjust to the compromises PD requires.

In some families, the partner of the person with PD takes the role of caregiver also. Peggy occupies this intermittently difficult position of being both partner and caregiver. In many situations and interactions, the two roles are mutually supportive. In others, conflict arises.

In many partnerships (and marriages), couples look for and work towards a balance. Many responsibilities are shared. Some are divided in an agreed upon arrangement. Accommodations occur. Despite stress and some imbalance, many partnerships flourish. Some continue a long time with mutual care, affection, love, and respect.

In some partnerships, one person will develop Parkinson's. Once Parkinson's develops and advances, balances become very hard to establish and maintain.

When a person takes on the role of caregiver of a partner, the established living patterns may change substantially. Many old balances are disturbed and disrupted. In solid relationships, each person feels that putting himself or herself first on a regular, frequent basis is acceptable. But when one partner becomes a caregiver the legitimacy may be questioned by both the caregiving partner and the partner with Parkinson's. Feeling that one should or is expected to "come second" all or most of the time, can cause a lot of resentment.

Also, someone who previously lived with a balance in giving and receiving may find the adjustment to giving more and receiving less very difficult and painful.

Simply taking on more work and responsibility may cause the partner-caregiver to feel overburdened and very tired. Sometimes, the partner-caregiver will feel absorbed by the illness.

One way of restoring some of the pre-Parkinson's balance includes spreading some caregiving responsibilities out among other family members and close friends.

Hiring a professional caregiver part-time or full-time may bring some balance back to the relationship.

With or without caregiving help, the partner-caregiver needs and deserves a lot of emotional support. Support groups for partner-caregivers offer an excellent safehaven for validation, understanding, and compassion.

Each of these ways of giving help to the partner-caregiver may enable the caregiver to return to feeling like a person with his or her own life.

In contrast to some other major diseases, people with PD rarely die of Parkinson's. Instead, they become progressively more disabled. The practical consequence of the nonfatal aspect of PD is that family caregivers must continue to function in their role for a very long period of time.

The relationship between the person with PD and the family caregiver is constantly changing as Parkinson's disease progresses. Previously, tasks done by the person with PD become more and more the responsibility of the family caregiver. As the person with PD becomes less self-sufficient and more dependent, the relationship, once built on equality, shifts in part, to a relationship between one person giving care and one receiving it. A great amount of patience, tact, and acceptance can help the relationship to maintain positive aspects and generate positive feelings.

While the person with PD often gets a lot of attention, family, friends, and medical personnel may ignore the difficulties of the partner caregiver role. Friends, family, and neighbors can quickly become tired of hearing about the caregiver's problems.

Many people with PD have the best of intentions, but they lose concentration and struggle or fail to complete an activity. Some caregivers find it easier to do the task themselves. The person with PD then may feel increasingly dependent and more frustrated and angry. To the person with PD, the inability to finish tasks or do more than one thing at a time can be very upsetting.

Conscious of the increased burdens placed on the family caregiver, some people with PD will still try to perform tasks that are now considered to be dangerous. The danger arises from their reduced sense of balance, their lack of mobility, and their slowed reaction times.

The question of whether the person with PD is able to help around the house safely also can cause arguments about what people with Parkinson's can and cannot do. The arguments force the person with PD and the caregiver to confront the increasing inability of the person to function independently as the illness progresses. The acknowledgment can produce anger and sorrow for both.

Some people with Parkinson's disease use their illness to get their way. They will cite their disabilities as an excuse to avoid doing chores around the house that they find odious. It is often difficult for a caregiver to distinguish between what is possible and what is not possible.

People with Parkinson's receive a lot of attention for having PD. Such attention can feel very good. Seeming helpless can bring more attention. With this reinforcement, the person with PD copes less well than his/her stage of Parkinson's might suggest. Further, the extra attention given to the person with PD really does not compensate for his/her loss of autonomy and influence in the family.

The power relationship is constantly changing as the caregiver becomes more assertive and the person with PD more dependent. The change creates a lot of stress and conflict.

Parkinson's presents many challenges to Peggy. She feels confusion, anger and a lot of stress at times. Still, she often responds by becoming more independent and flexible. She feels she can cope better with responsibilities. Her overall functioning is better. She is taking a leadership role in the family.

Family caretakers often complain that as Parkinson's disease progresses, people with PD become more self-centered and less sensitive to the partner and the rest of the family. People with serious, chronic illnesses often do not recognize their self-absorption. They feel surprised and often angry when it is brought to their attention. I remembered Peggy's confronting me one afternoon. I had been going through a particularly intense period of introspection. She said that I was not paying sufficient attention to her, that I wasn't helping around the house, and that I was very hyperactive and also distant. As usual, my first reaction to these kinds of comments was to become angry, defensive, and attacking while denying these attitudes and behaviors.

My surprise at Peggy's statements was genuine. From my perspective, I had been especially attentive. However, Peggy made clear that I can and do shut out people sometimes while being totally unaware of my behavior. I do not like this aspect of myself, nor do I like being reminded of it. To her credit, Peggy brought all of this behavior to my attention. She was fully knowledgeable of the storm that would follow.

After a lot of defensive maneuvering, some attacks, and some exaggerated justifications, I began to see that Peggy had a point. I had not been paying enough attention to the person who loved me, helped me, and extended her efforts for me beyond the ordinary range.

Parkinson's is a heavy burden. How much is this negative behavior a result of Parkinson's? Is the tendency toward self-centeredness inevitable or can I overcome it? We all need to think and talk about these questions.

My wife was understandably worried about how the rhythms of our life together would change. Parkinson's results in profound changes for the partner that are almost as big as those for the person with PD. Because PD is progressive, the relationship and problems between the person with PD and the partner constantly are changing. Peggy feels that she regularly has to adjust to a different me. She longs for the pre-Parkinson's days. I worry that I am going to exhaust those near and dear to me.

Many problems occur on a more mundane level. Dressing presents a real challenge. Summer's humidity adds to my frustration and causes me to need more help. Opening plastic bags can be particularly difficult because of perceptual problems. To be on time for an activity, a person with PD and the caregiver must force themselves to start getting ready much earlier than before the development of PD.

People with PD often speak softly and trail off at the end of sentences. They are mostly unaware of this behavior. It is not unusual for friends and partners to say "I can't hear you" or "I heard all but the last word."

My talking to Peggy from another room and talking quietly has been the source of numerous discussions. My quiet speech and the friction it causes are among some of the constant irritants associated with PD.

Empathy and support provide a floor for the person with PD and the partner to make a good life after the diagnosis. Expressions of appreciation and efforts to be independent can foster a good relationship between the person with Parkinson's and the partner. Living in an engaged and connected manner contributes greatly to the quality of life together. As always, talking about problems can bring better understanding. With many interpersonal problems, professional help often can be beneficial.

Good communication between people with Parkinson's disease and their partners enables them to work together on the problems PD causes and to enjoy their lives. Poor communication makes a lot of life much harder.

Part of the solution to communication issues involves agreement on what each person can and will try to do to make communication easier. We have found that being in the same room when we want to talk makes hearing and understanding much easier.

The effort to go to the partner before talking may be stressful or take extra time. Still, walking before talking really enhances communication and avoids a lot of tension and frustration. For some, movement is or becomes too much of a challenge. Then, some couples may want to use a whistle for calling for attention or help or an intercom for an actual conversation.

When talking, couples can rely on a few principles to make their feelings and their ideas clear. No person can hear or see the thoughts of another. Therefore, no person can assume correctly that someone else understands her/him without clear statements or questions and sufficient details. When one person speaks his/her feelings about the listener, the comments can be received best when they begin with "I feel" rather than with "you did," or "you made," or "you" with some other verb as accusation or blame. Listening after talking is part of a conversation. Finally, sometimes saying less is more effective for getting a satisfying response.

Parkinson's disease puts extreme stress on relationships within the family. Family members will need to adjust to many changes in their relationships with the person who has PD and, at times, with each other.

These changes and the stresses they cause can make family members angry at the person who has Parkinson's disease. In many households, anger remains under some control. Sometimes, a lot of anger develops and is repressed or suppressed. Subsequently, an angry outburst may occur, such as an adolescent or even an adult tantrum. The outburst releases emotional pressure, but sometimes no resolution of the conflict occurs.

People with Parkinson's and their families need to recognize the power of anger and try to express it constructively. Developing coping mechanisms for their own anger and in reaction to the anger of others will lead to better self-acceptance and better family relationships.

Mutual patience, tolerance, and support can help ease tensions within the family. Sometimes, professional help can benefit everyone involved. Participation in a support group can provide an accepting and nurturing atmosphere for coping with the powerful emotions evoked when trying to cope with this intrusive and demanding disease. Counseling or therapy for individual family members, the couple, or the family as a unit can be very helpful.

Partly because of the demands and great stresses arising from PD, family members can be insensitive, ignorant, rude, and hostile to people who have Parkinson's disease. Some family members may be distressed openly by tremors or other symptoms. Others may be uncomfortable with the amount of attention given when family members take the time for a person with

Parkinson's disease to act by her/himself individually and with friends and in pleasurable activities.

Many people with Parkinson's feel a special concern about their children. If the children are still quite young, explaining PD to them requires an approach tailored to their age and ability to understand and accept illness and disability. Having a parent with Parkinson's will bring sorrow to any child no matter the age. Because of the loss of some attention, companionship, and help, some children of any age will feel both sad and angry. Older children, including adult children, will feel anxiety about both the parent's future and their own as it is tied to the parent's. At some point, children will worry about their own health, especially whether they too will develop PD.

Providing the children opportunities to talk and encouraging a sharing of feelings between parents and children will help maintain and perhaps even enhance the relationships.

Our own children, Andrew and Joanna, have remained concerned and caring. They both reached adulthood before Parkinson's Disease attacked. Therefore, their understanding of the illness has been very thorough. They feel sorrow about the limitations and disabilities that PD has been inflicting on me. They also feel very sad that PD has limited what I can enjoy with them. Andrew and Joanna both experience my having Parkinson's as a loss for me and for them. In their individual ways, they have expressed their love through many different efforts and gestures of help and companionship over the years I have struggled with Parkinson's. We are very grateful for and enjoy very much their love and involvement.

Our son-in-law, Aaron Harsh serves as my computer consultant and tech. He helps in many other ways too.

Our grandchildren have been concerned and helpful as well. At first, our grandson, Derek, stood and looked at me closely. He announced that he was checking me out! Every once in a while, Derek asks me how my Parkinson's is. As he matures, he tries to help me as much as possible. He has stopped me from falling many times.

Although younger, our grand-daughter, Asia has been helpful as well. She is very eager to open doors and push me in my transport chair.

All of the children and grandchildren have been concerned about the difficulty in predicting what will happen as Parkinson's disease progresses. For these concerns, one cannot give clear answers.

CHAPTER 3

Parkinson's Disease and the Community

The sociologist Ferdinand Tönnies drew a distinction between early rural communities and modern market-dominated communities. The early communities were relatively simple. Their values supported the strength and success of the group rather than the welfare of the individual. They felt that the function of the community included caring for its members to ensure the survival of the group. Individual rights were not emphasized. As with market-dominated communities, social control was the responsibility of law enforcement, the neighborhood, education, religion, and the family. There was neither social nor economic mobility. An individual did not move from one social class to another. Therefore, a person was secure in her/his place. The interpersonal relationships were called primary. Community residents knew each other in many capacities. By contrast, in modern society, people tend to know each other through a specific role. This type of relationship is considered secondary. It is less encompassing than a primary relationship.

Beyond help within the family, the provision of social services for those in need was seen as a residual function carried out mostly by volunteers. However, as capitalism replaced feudalism, roles became more specialized. In the process, the family gradually lost some of its supporting and caretaking functions. Formal public, private, and religious organizations began to provide programs for the disabled and the poor.

Most funding decisions became and still are predominantly political decisions. There was and remains resistance to government funding of social welfare programs. Usually the most politically powerful groups received and still do receive the most funding.

American society has been organized in part around the principle of survival of the fittest. This principle supports the idea that each person should make his/her own way and take care of himself/herself. It asserts that society gains when the strong survive and prosper.

Exceptions to survival of the fittest can be found within certain religious, ethnic, and social groups and some individuals. Exceptions in governmental policies occurred during the Great Depression in the 1930s and during the War on Poverty in the 1960s.

Today, this attitude of individuals being responsible only for themselves prevails over the value of group responsibility for all of its members. It explains in part why poor, sick, disabled, and mentally ill people often do not get the help and respect they deserve and need. The needs and rights of ethnic and racial minorities and women also have been ignored because of the attitude that those who do well have no responsibility for those who don't.

Throughout my social work career in Milwaukee, I took an active role in community issues. Through teaching many students, conducting research, and working with others on committees, giving speeches, speaking to the press, writing editorials and two books, and supporting candidates for public office, I devoted a lot of time, energy, and expertise in efforts to make Milwaukee a better place to live for the poor & disabled.

I found working with community leaders to be both effective and stimulating. I met many interesting and dedicated people. I feel that I was able to influence some public policies. When my Parkinson's disease became more debilitating, I needed to give up some of these activities.

Finally, I resigned from the community boards, stopped conducting new research, and ultimately retired from teaching. Parkinson's disease forced me to withdraw from the academic community and the community of Milwaukeeans working to influence public policy.

For people with Parkinson's disease, giving up activities and memberships in various organizations and groups can lead to feelings of isolation. A withdrawal of interest in the surrounding world may follow eventually. To try to avoid isolation, some people with PD may choose to join new groups and organizations more in tune with their changing interests and capacities.

CHAPTER 4

Going Public: Communicating about One's Parkinson's Disease

For a person who has developed PD, one difficult decision concerns whether, when, and how to tell family, friends, and colleagues. Many relatives, friends, and work colleagues already will have noticed that the person with Parkinson's disease walks differently, seems stiff, and has trouble dressing. The voice may be soft. In general, the person with PD will seem different. In short, any announcement of the illness may tell others what they already know.

Even though one may want to ignore the fact of having PD, persistent symptoms will make this effort difficult. The need to tell others about having PD may occur before one has integrated the reality of the disease. A double burden exists in coping with one's own feelings about having PD while at the same time announcing the medical problems to others.

Eventually, many people with PD feel a need to tell others that they have developed PD. As with so many things in life, there is no one way to announce that one has a serious illness. The popular phrase "different strokes for different folks" is a good guideline.

After talking with a significant other or close friend, one needs to decide what one is going to say to whom.

One might start out with a relatively simple and short description about PD. Family and friends do want some basic knowledge about PD, including how it will affect their relationship with the person who has Parkinson's disease and what activities will become too difficult or impossible.

Telling other people about being ill with Parkinson's disease can be difficult and stressful. Telling family members, friends, and colleagues takes careful thought. Whom to tell and how much to tell should be based in part on the closeness of the relationship. It is important to remember that people without Parkinson's may not be as interested in the details of the illness. The listener probably will make clear how much he/she wants to know. Deciding how much to tell depends also on the age and the sensitivity of the listener. Adults can understand and integrate much more information than children. Determining how much to reveal at the place of employment depends on how secure and how competitive one's position is. Another factor concerns the degree of illness. The person with Parkinson's should consider whether and when his or her symptoms will affect job performance. This information may be shared or withheld.

Talking with children may be especially difficult. Older children might have noticed that their parent frequently loses balance or that the tension in the household has risen since the parent developed PD. Mostly, children are concerned with PD's effects on their lives. Experiencing and talking about a parent having PD may be especially hard for teenagers because they are extremely concerned about their image. They may feel that having an obviously ill parent reflects badly on them. Issues of separation also may be extremely difficult for teenagers because they are struggling to become more independent while their parent is becoming more dependent.

One should limit one's own talking so that enough time remains for questions. Saying one does not know the answer to a specific question is both honest and acceptable. Some questions, like "how long can one function normally?" are unanswerable. The door should always remain open for future discussions about PD.

Informing others whom one knows well causes the news to spread. One also might receive unhelpful or poorly informed suggestions and comments. Yet others seem to have a special sense of when to offer help and when to let me continue on my own. Once I thought I would fall down while trying to sit in a restaurant chair. My friend quickly appeared from his place at the table to help me. He showed empathy and was discrete. Other friends and colleagues have asked how I am and often hugged me. Others just want reassurance that I am all right. Still others seem to feel very uncomfortable and awkward. The way in which they relate robs me of my wholeness and suggests they see me primarily as a sick person.

A typical conversation might sound like this:

"Hello, Bob. How are you feeling?"

"I am feeling good. Thanks for asking."

"But how are you doing?"

"I am on new medication, and it is working very well."

"Well, good to see you, Bob. Take care. Good-bye."

When I first talked about having Parkinson's disease, I resented others' focus on my illness. Perhaps I was still trying to deny it, or I just didn't want to have PD as a main topic of my time with friends. It is not necessary to talk about it at length, but PD cannot be ignored. I have come to realize that most people are genuinely concerned, and, inevitably, having Parkinson's has become part of my identity.

In my case, I struggled with whether I should tell my students. I talked to colleagues and friends about it and received differing opinions. I finally decided that my symptoms were becoming obvious, and my students lack of knowledge about PD was worse than talking with them about my disease. When I made my announcement, I discovered that many students already knew I had PD! Some were interested in how PD would affect the class.

Some students didn't seem to care as long as I could function adequately as a teacher. A few students asked some questions, such as whether I would continue teaching (yes) and what was on the midterm! Some students came up after class and were sympathetic.

Since my voice was weak, I had the university furnish me with a microphone so I could be heard clearly. Overall, the experience was anticlimactic.

Some people feel very uncomfortable about asking for and receiving help. Many people with PD need some help but like to remain as independent as possible. Issues to consider are how to ask for help, how to accept help, under what conditions, and when and how to refuse help.

I remember an evening when I tripped out of a restaurant. Immediately the people who were waiting to be seated came to my assistance. A man grabbed me around the waist. A woman put her shoulders under one of my arms. A teenager grabbed the back of my coat. They worked to pull me back onto my feet.

Sometimes too many people try to help. Occasionally, their efforts are counterproductive. Their efforts can confuse me and, ultimately, fail. Often, my wife asserts herself and chooses one person to help on one side of me while she helps on the other side.

CHAPTER 5

Parkinson's Disease and Mental Health

As a progressive illness, Parkinson's disease can have a powerful effect on the mental health of people who live with it. When my neurologist announced that I had Parkinson's, he confirmed what I suspected but had tried to suppress. Acknowledging my illness altered my life completely. The rest of my life has been a process of adapting as I try to fight this chronic disease.

One never totally adjusts to continuous change. PD has a major effect on all aspects of my life. I have gone through a series of adjustments that have affected my personality and my relationships with friends and family.

Parkinson's stirs up many strong emotions. What is best, expression or suppression? Is it best to talk about the illness and try to integrate it into daily life or not to talk and try to keep all the emotion, especially anger, inside? I have had to deal with a large amount of anger toward myself and my body and others who don't have PD and who don't understand what I am going through. I wonder why I have Parkinson's disease and not someone else. Life seems unfair. Thinking about some of the activities that I now find difficult or can no longer do makes me sad. Thinking about the future can make me feel very anxious.

Having Parkinson's disease can be a very emotional experience. Anger develops from frustration, loss, needing help, and feeling restricted and controlled. It is hard to imagine someone with PD who is not angry about having the disease.

For me, PD has produced a lot of anger of which I am not always aware. I am basically a gentle, supportive, positive individual who tries to avoid conflict. But every once in a while, my underlying anger about Parkinson's and perhaps other aspects of my life bursts through. I become hostile. I sometimes don't think before I talk. I am capable of saying mean and hurtful things. I feel anger can be a normal response to living with a difficult illness.

I apologize and try to understand what is happening. The anger may be unprovoked. My anger, while in specific incidents focuses on specific individuals, is really quite generalized.

Some people express their anger openly. Such open expressions of anger can be quite healthy. Problems can arise if the anger grows out of control and the angry person becomes physically or emotionally abusive.

On the other hand, some people turn their anger inward and become depressed. Controlled open expressions of anger can help both the person with the feelings of anger and the person to whom the angry feelings are directed.

For various reasons, significant others, children, family, friends, and caregivers can become angry at the person with PD. People with PD are different from the way they used to be. They often make more extensive demands than they did before they developed PD. Their capacity to contribute to the lives they share changes and diminishes. Anger from their families and friends surprises some people with PD. They may feel they are coping well. They often are not aware of how much they have changed or how much help they need. They may not be aware of how much loss their family and friends are experiencing. Further, wives, husbands, partners, children, and friends can be embarrassed about the behavior and appearance of their loved one. Their embarrassment also can generate anger.

Having to wait for the help they need, people with PD sometimes become angry with others. They may direct their anger toward family and friends who struggle to cope with personal needs as well as the needs of the person with PD.

The increased level of tension and the difficulty in satisfying everyone's needs may contribute to family members' and family caregivers' angry outbursts or anger simmering beneath the surface. These feelings, when unresolved, can work against positive, loving relationships. Good relationships can be weakened, and weak relationships can be put at further risk.

It is important for communication about feelings to be maintained. I had no idea, for example, of the degree to which my illness was affecting my wife. Uncomfortable with her own feelings, she did not share them with me at first.

All people are responsible for their own feelings and behavior. It is how people decide to express and cope with their feelings in words and behavior which determines how they get along with each other.

Anger can be displaced. Spouses can be blamed for conflicts with children even though they are not involved in the conflict. A famous Norman Rockwell cartoon in an old *The Saturday Evening Post* showed a series of drawings in which anger was displaced. In the first picture, an employer criticized his employee. In the next picture, the employee yelled at his wife. Then the wife got mad at her son. Finally, the son yelled at the dog! The original anger was displaced, ultimately, to the dog, an innocent victim.

Anger can also be very destructive. Words spoken in a moment of anger may last a lifetime. Even short-lived anger may affect negatively feelings and actions of the people involved well into the future.

People with Parkinson's disease need to acknowledge and appreciate the help that their support system is providing. People with PD who feel guilty about needing help should recognize and understand the guilt.

Otherwise, anger about feeling guilty can become anger at the helpers.

Expressing and discussing anger can be productive because both help people to clarify and understand each other's positions. Expressing upset feelings can relieve emotional pressure. An airing of feelings can help people to work toward a resolution of conflicts or to continue struggling with the difficult problems that arise from living with PD. Professional counselors or therapists can help people with PD and members of their support network find ways to talk about their feelings and cope with them.

Perhaps one reason for the anger is the hostility in American society toward those who cannot take adequate care of themselves. Dependency can be a negative word, and most people do not want to be dependent or to be considered dependent. Many people tend to "blame the victim" of Parkinson's and other mental and physical disabilities. Charles Darwin's concept of "survival of the fittest" has influenced the thinking of many people. Many people in the past and today make small and large, personal and public decisions based on the idea that only people who live without assistance and special accommodations should survive. The Social Darwinists believe that people should be expected to cope on their own. They feel that outside support for the poor, the sick and those with mental health problems weakens the society.

Impatience often accompanies Parkinson's disease. People with PD often become impatient with family, friends, and others in their surrounding environment. Many also become impatient with themselves. The impatience, slowness, and growing dependency can lead to family, friends, and others frequently feeling intolerant of a person with PD.

On a more basic level, people with Parkinson's disease may lose independence, feelings of self-reliance, and confidence in their bodies. They may lose a sense of being reliable and dependable. They no longer may feel comfortable being outside their own homes.

The lack of mobility, which occurs for many people who have Parkinson's disease, can be devastating and can affect almost all aspects of life. Taken for granted by most of the population, a loss of mobility is a serious problem.

Many people with Parkinson's must give up physical activities they have loved. It can be very difficult to maintain activities that require a lot of endurance, balance, and flexibility. Many people with PD may need to stop hiking, driving an automobile, participating in sports, and traveling.

Losses can lead to sorrow, grief, and depression. For many, expressing the sorrow, grief, and depression that can stem from great loss may help with learning to live within new parameters. People with PD should be allowed to grieve without the pressure to "snap out of it" or to stop "indulging in self-pity." By acknowledging and accepting these feelings, caregivers, spouses, significant others, family, and friends can offer comfort and acceptance.

Being labeled as a disabled person can have further negative consequences for someone's sense of self. The label affects interactions between the labeler and the person with PD. Being treated as different, incompetent, or helpless can make a person feel like an inadequate and very dependent outsider.

When I first developed Parkinson's disease, I felt very isolated. Then I discovered that Parkinson's disease is much more prevalent than I had realized. Some of my friends have PD. Many of them have friends and relatives who have Parkinson's disease. While I still feel isolated at times, having empathic help and support from others makes a difference. Over time, as the burdens of Parkinson's increase, it is helpful to try to maintain a positive outlook on life.

It is difficult to explain the subtle changes in emotion and behavior over time that affect many people with

Parkinson's. The early years with PD may not be very difficult. For many, the illness worsens gradually. However, just as a person with PD feels able to cope with one symptom, another appears. This advance of symptoms can lead to frustration, upset, and anger.

More advanced symptoms of PD are not subtle at all. Rigid muscles throughout the body, shuffling, inability to speak clearly or to eat without help all can become a part of daily life. Falling in the house or on neighborhood streets can bring bruises, frustration, and embarrassment.

Often, people with Parkinson's wonder about the relationship between their minds and their bodies. Can their thoughts and desires overcome their physical limitations? Can people with PD exercise and go to physical therapy enough to overcome some of their disabilities? Are people with Parkinson's to blame if they don't improve their functioning? Everyone has heard stories of individuals who survive deadly diseases like cancer. Everyone has heard as well of those who die prematurely even though they appear to be healthy. Perhaps what can be said is that a positive attitude and an effort to comply with treatment, such as taking medicine on schedule and exercising and doing physical therapy homework cannot hurt future functioning. But it is a heavy burden for those suffering from PD to be considered responsible for not doing better.

When I first was diagnosed with Parkinson's disease, I found myself walking around and looking at people who appeared normal. Why do some people have some diseases and others do not? Many want to know exactly what caused their illness. Some question whether they are being punished for their sins. Some ask if they can blame their parents' genes. Some wonder if years of walking a dog exposed them to a lot of pollution. I ask if my lifelong interest in photography exposed me to toxic chemicals. I probably never will know the answer.

People with Parkinson's know that the disease is progressive and can be extremely disabling. This knowledge puts extra pressure on the person with PD who often is driven by the desire to do a lot of living before he or she becomes incapacitated. This desire is true of all of us to some extent. We all age, and some of us become less competent. But the tumble into dependency seems more poignant, visible, and pervasive than the normal process of aging. What develops is a more frantic feeling as medication becomes less effective and creates disturbing side effects.

CHAPTER 6

The Early Stages of Parkinson's Disease

For a long time after being diagnosed with Parkinson's disease, I felt desperate. Desperation led to an intense effort to understand the disease and, hopefully, to control it. I tried to obtain all the information I could. I talked with my neurologist. I downloaded many studies from the Internet. I clipped newspaper and magazine articles and read a number of books by people with Parkinson's disease. I went to conferences about PD. My friends and relatives sent me clippings that documented new approaches to controlling the PD symptoms.

After all my research, I felt I had only a beginner's understanding of the disease. "Parkinson's disease may be one of the more baffling and complex of all neurological disorders" (Nauseida and Bock, "Parkinson Disease: What You and Your Family Should Know" The Network September, 2000, p. 7). "It is one of a continuum of neurological disorders whose causes are uncertain and for which there are no known cures (ibid., 3)."

Understanding Parkinson's disease became a full-time job and the main focus of my life. Friends and family, especially my wife, felt shut out. Because no one could say how long I would be functioning adequately, I became obsessive in my effort to get my affairs in order.

Peggy and I reviewed our will, our investments, and our insurance policies. We talked about adding a bathroom on the first floor. For a month, I searched for the perfect file cabinet for my papers and lecture materials. I spent another two months reading all my papers and filing the ones I wanted to keep. I began to clean the basement and attic and to reorganize the garage. I improved my home office and bought a more powerful computer so I could work on our book. I acted like a constant whirlwind. I swept through my family, oblivious to anything in my way.

During that time, teaching became a major challenge. I found myself tremoring sometimes during my lectures. I had trouble projecting my voice. I sometimes went to class struggling to think clearly. At times I could not teach for longer than two hours. Often, I dismissed the class early so I could go home and collapse.

I became less social and resented the concern from others over my condition. Because of a very low energy level, I deliberately missed many meetings at the university. Fatigue led to my cutting back on my community activities and resigning from the boards of two community social agencies. Retirement became necessary three and a half years after my diagnosis.

During this early period, medication changes came frequently. My doctor made adjustments to determine the most effective dosages of the most effective medications. Major changes required allowing the previous medication to wash out of the body before a new medication could be started. Functioning with too little or no medication for even a short while created a lot of discomfort, an increase in some symptoms, and great anxiety. The biggest problem was the sense of loss of control over my body and my life. This feeling became especially intense when changing medication required a confining hospital stay.

Each time I adjusted to the new medication regimen, I could see clearly the importance of Parkinson's medication in coping effectively with PD. I began to feel much better. My sleep and walking improved, and I froze less often. I was more related to my family, my friends, and myself.

Because Parkinson's disease is progressive, physicians may make periodic changes to medication. Therefore, people with PD should keep their scheduled medical appointments and make additional ones when they feel the need.

CHAPTER 7

Coping with Chronic Disability

I know people who are trying to cope with PD by taking only a little or no medication. They are gambling that in the long run, by delaying taking medication, they will have a long period without serious physical and cognitive side effects. For some people, delaying the use of medication works out best. For others, wisdom lies in beginning medication early in the course of the illness. People with PD should make this decision in consultation with their physicians.

Hopefully, new medicines will be developed that will lessen the side effects and maintain effectiveness even with long-term use. To choose a medication that may help now but lead to functioning less well at some future date can feel like a dangerous decision. I have chosen to take my medicine now and deal with any consequences later. This decision feels acceptable, but the possibility of future difficulties disturbs me.

I stopped driving a car because of depth perception and judgment problems. Then I stopped riding my bicycle because of my increasingly insecure sense of balance. After falling off my bike and nearly being hit by a car, I became frightened of riding. I thought my bicycle-riding days had ended. However, my son, Andrew, an avid bicycle rider, suggested I ride a three-wheeler. The third wheel ensures stability. The three-wheelers are fun to ride and for me are more comfortable than a regular bicycle.

When I went for a test ride, the salesman let me take the three-wheeler outside. I had a great time and was convinced that my bike-riding days were being revived. I was so excited that I told the salesman that I had PD and had very bad balance and that he and the bike store had made my return to bike riding possible.

The atmosphere changed immediately. The salesman started to talk about sickness. He was less relaxed, and I thought he related to me as a sick, handicapped person. I was jolted into reality. I remembered that I was different, and that in many social situations, my Parkinson's symptoms were there for the entire world to see. I did not realize that I had introduced the subject of disability and thus may have triggered the salesman's change in attitude.

Most PD patients stand out in some way whether by gait, tremors, canes, or walkers. It is hard to be anonymous with Parkinson's. What people with Parkinson's want is first to have their disability recognized quietly. Then they want others to see beyond the disability to the whole person.

Even with a multifaceted sense of self, people with PD can find maintaining a positive outlook very difficult as the disease progresses. PD can be depressing. The disease certainly makes daily living difficult.

When others focus on only the disability, the label *disabled* can become the determinant of the whole identity of people with PD. Being seen only as a person with Parkinson's can have negative consequences for one's self-confidence. While there are a range of adaptations people make to Parkinson's disease, all people with PD are affected emotionally. The brains of people with PD do not manufacture the needed amount of dopamine. Because low levels of dopamine can result in depression, astute physicians will prescribe an antidepressant for some of their patients with PD.

There may be periods when the disease does not progress. For some, there can be a period of life when their symptoms do not worsen. However, for many, the times of relative peace are finite.

According to the actor Michael J. Fox, who has Parkinson's disease, "It [Parkinson's] changes you, this disease. And I've discovered a certain level of surrender to it, which isn't to say capitulation or allowing it to overwhelm me. Surrendering can mean a certain level of acceptance of the limitations Parkinson's disease determines (FOX, AARP, 2006, p64)."

I have reached the point, to some extent, of recognizing and accepting my limitations. This acceptance is an ongoing process. I no longer can do a lot of things that I used to do. I am becoming more able to accept the kindness of strangers.

Parkinson's is not the only disease whose symptoms call attention to the ill person. People with other illnesses and disabilities also receive stares. People who struggle with Parkinson's disease need to express their upset and to have empathic friends, relatives, and medical professionals. People with PD sometimes need to be reminded to focus on what they want to do rather than on the rudeness and insensitivity of others.

Getting adequate sleep can be a serious problem. Many people with Parkinson's need extra sleep. I almost have fallen asleep while talking to someone. Nearly falling asleep occurred not because of being bored, but because I did not sleep the night before. Public performances—plays, films, and concerts—are all cultural events I enjoy. Sometimes I miss parts because of my tendency to doze. This tendency to get drowsy unexpectedly can be dangerous, especially if one is driving a car or operating machinery.

Sleeping well is a challenge. While falling asleep at the wrong time is a problem, not falling asleep at the right time is frustrating. Tightness of the arms and legs is common and can interfere with relaxation and sleep.

Even without muscle tightness, relaxing can be difficult. I sometimes have had trouble sleeping if I have wine, beer, or chocolate or anything else containing caffeine for supper. I have spent many nights unable to relax into sleep. I have tried to read a novel, watch TV, go downstairs to the kitchen to get a snack, edit my manuscript, often to no avail.

There are several approaches that can help alleviate the problem of insomnia. A good massage from a significant other can help one to relax and relieve the muscle pain sometimes associated with PD. I have found that doing yoga stretching for ten or fifteen minutes can help me to relax. Sometimes watching a boring TV program helps to induce sleep. Taking a warm bath, reading a book, or drinking decaffeinated tea or warm milk also are possibilities.

Occasionally, I have very active dreams. I can make loud noises and flail on the bed. I usually don't remember the episodes in the morning. Needless to say, they are very disturbing to Peggy and me. My doctor says these eruptions are typical of people with PD.

It is hard to explain the terror of not being able to get a good night's sleep to those who do not have this problem. Not sleeping well often means that my Parkinson's symptoms—freezing, shuffling, loss of balance, and taking tiny rapid steps—are worse. The rest of the family worry about me and are understandably resentful when I wake them up during the night.

I know that if I stay up too many consecutive nights, I am going to develop a bad habit of sleeping during the day and working during the night. This pattern is great for book writing but awful for having a social life.

For a long time, I was having troubles focusing my eyes, especially when I was very tired and had spent a lot of time reading or looking at the computer screen. My optometrist prescribed reading glasses with prisms to help me focus. Using these glasses has made reading much easier. The proper prescription may help a lot.

Some people with PD are unable to remain full-time on their jobs. Others must retire after working for most of their adult lives. They are abruptly severed from the world of work. They struggle to cope with both PD and the loss of work. They may feel useless, alienated, and unable to find activities they enjoy. For some, the shift in role from a position of high status and authority at work to someone who doesn't have enough interests and energy to fill up a day can be painful. They feel peripheral to the general flow of life. They can become needy and difficult to live with.

At some point in the course of the illness, the family may feel a need for a designated family caregiver or a professional one. Of course, not all caregivers are spouses or significant others. Individuals with no relationship to the family can be hired to assist or to take partial or total care of the person with PD. Hiring a professional caregiver can give time to the spouse to work, do errands, and enjoy chosen activities.

Hiring a caregiver can be expensive. Sometimes there are personality conflicts. Some people resist having an outsider come into their home. Some can be suspicious of the honesty of an outside caregiver and resist change.

Also difficult are thinking and talking about Parkinson's disease. Both the person with PD and the family members may struggle to communicate their feelings. Many people with Parkinson's disease find it easier not to talk about it. Eventually, many people with PD feel the need to discuss the implications of having a progressive illness. Such a time may become an opportunity to talk about feelings.

Since both Peggy and I have been professional social workers and partners in coping with Parkinson's disease, we support the approach of talking openly and getting appropriate outside help when family and friends can't help. In general, talking about the effect of PD on our marriage has been useful. We have had rough times when the short-term effects of talking about PD have not been as positive as we had hoped. In the long run, we feel talk is best, even considering how uncomfortable it can be.

With whom should one talk about coping with Parkinson's a spouse, a good friend, a trusted religious advisor, or a human service professional? Some people are more comfortable talking with a trusted religious advisor about their PD problems while others feel most comfortable going to professional counselors. Some people rely on family and friends. In any event, the issues do not go away automatically and, ultimately, have to be faced.

Having Parkinson's takes a lot of work. A person with Parkinson's disease needs to schedule time for stretching to keep his/her muscles loose. People with PD need to remember to take their medication at the right time. Getting enough exercise is essential. There are so many daily routines! Almost any activity takes more time than it formerly did.

Like so many others, I am tired of having a chronic illness. Periodically, participating actively in my care becomes too difficult. Sometimes depression interferes with my self-help routines. However, for me, there is no viable alternative to struggling. I am thankful to be functioning as well as I do. I have been lucky so far that my Parkinson's disease has been controlled, to a large extent, by excellent medical care and medication. Also contributing to keeping my symptoms under control are exercise, sufficient rest, and my determination to persist despite embarrassment and periodic failure. Enjoying life as much as possible is key to coping well.

People with Parkinson's may have times when their symptoms are minor, and they cope very well. Having periods of functioning very well does not mean the disease is cured. In the past, I sometimes became cocky and felt that I did not need to take my medication all the time. I believed that I had conquered the disease and that my doctor would feel quite proud of me. Then, I would feel my legs tighten up. My PD shuffle returned. My balance would deteriorate. I would break out into a cold sweat. One of the times these sensations put me in a panicky state. Needing help, I called the Parkinson's clinic. The nurse said that if I didn't take my medication, my symptoms would overtake me. The statement was clear and logical. But the desire to be free of Parkinson's disease and the pain had blocked my ability to think and act rationally.

CONCLUSION

Parkinson's disease can be an all-encompassing disease. It affects the mind, the body and the spirit.

For those who have Parkinson's, fighting the disease can be very challenging. A symptom might disappear temporarily only to be replaced by a different symptom. Experiencing multiple symptoms requires solving multiple problems sometimes at once.

It should be noted that not all people experience every symptom. In addition, the intensity of the symptoms can vary from one individual to the next.

Some experts feel that Parkinson's is a number of different diseases with similar characteristics but different etiologies. "Inheritance of certain genes, environmental pollution, and traumatic assaults to the brain" (Hyde 2011) are some of the factors being focused on as causes of PD.

Some people have hallucinations as a side effect of the medication they must take to combat Parkinson's disease. In a hallucination, individuals will see people and/or animals who actually are not present. Sometimes their "presence" is quite time limited. They usually remain silent. Their appearance may cause anxiety and avoidance in the person with Parkinson's. Explaining the existence of hallucinations as a product of the Parkinson's-affected brain doesn't always eliminate the feeling of the person with PD that the hallucinations are real. Reassurance that they are harmless may be a comfort.

Mobility, important in the modern world, is limited or absent for many people with Parkinson's. Because people with Parkinson's are not very mobile, they may be cut off from a wide variety of social and economic activities. PD has destroyed relationships, friendships, and self-esteem.

What is one going to do for the rest of one's life as one slowly becomes more dependent, less competent, and more uncomfortable? For those who have had a rich and vigorous life, the slow slide into dependency can be devastating.

As life slows down and one's focus narrows, the opportunity arises to pay attention and enjoy the small things in life—the beauty of wildflowers, the dew on farmland in the morning, and the human-made beauties of two and three dimensional art.

Planning one's life becomes very difficult. Many people with PD share a constant concern. They worry they will not be able to complete everything they want to do and experience before their disability completely stops their efforts. People with Parkinson's benefit from working around the limits set by the disease and finally accepting the limits that cannot be transcended. Benefits come from doing what they can to enjoy life and to contribute to the lives of others. Avoiding a retreat into the safety of home and pushing oneself to socialize with friends and to get out into the community are important. Treasuring loved ones is crucial.

One needs to be courageous to live with Parkinson's disease. People feel scared and depressed when told they have Parkinson's disease. They may look at themselves as dysfunctional and different and tend to withdraw. Every stage is disabling and can be traumatic. With PD one's mobility is diminished. One shakes in public. One risks freezing and falling. Basic activities such as crossing the street are more dangerous.

Some people with PD, rather than withdrawing, try to look outward. One can visit, e-mail, or telephone some friends. Connecting with others lifts one's mood. Going to see a film or renting a video expands one's thinking. Making a trip to a nearby art museum or sporting event expands one's experience and provides subjects to share with friends. Reading the newspaper is a way of staying informed about what is going on in the world.

To reduce feelings of isolation, one can become involved in a local Parkinson's support group. One can organize a support group if the community lacks one. Experts report that owning and taking care of an animal can relieve feelings of loneliness and reduces anxiety. The type of animal will determine how much care is needed.

In the article "Attitude," Dr. Gary Leo writes, "Parkinson Disease will disrupt your life. Parkinson will affect your family, your friends, and community. Just when you feel there is a let up new symptoms appear and adjustments are necessary (Leo 2010)."

The course of the disease is unpredictable, and planning for the future is challenging if not impossible. As Paul Mamerow, P.A.-C. says, "When you're hot, you're hot! When you're not, you're not!" (Mamerow 2011, from a song by Jerry Jeff Walker).

Advocacy plays an important role in helping people with PD. Michael J. Fox, the actor, is an example of a highly visible advocate who has advanced the country's understanding of Parkinson's disease. He has a special insight on Parkinson's based on his own experiences with PD. Fox has established a national foundation, The Michael J. Fox Foundation for Parkinson's Research. Fox supports political action as well. Another national leader in advocating for people with Parkinson's is Davis Phinney, who also has PD. He leads a foundation to promote exercise for living well with Parkinson's. Like Michael J. Fox, Davis Phinney takes a positive approach to PD. Phinney promotes exercise through his bike racing and bike rides. His foundation, The Davis Phinney Foundation emphasizes the power of the individual to cope with Parkinson's disease. Both Fox and Phinney advocate increasing private and governmental funding for research on PD.

The U.S. political system is dominated primarily by powerful private and public organizations. Those interested in developing policies supportive of people with Parkinson's need to develop skills to cope with the political nature of the American social welfare system. In many areas of mental and physical health, decisions are made that ignore relevant policy research. Without relevant and effective intervention in policy-making, destructive decisions can be made.

Health and social welfare provisions for PD are a mixture of outpatient medical care, inpatient medical care, family care, professional caregiving services, and long-term care facilities.

Despite the variety, these provisions remain inadequate. Many communities have no provisions beyond family care. What provisions exist outside the home are too expensive for many families. Little or no avenues for respite for family caregivers exist.

Exercise is very important. In Milwaukee, Susan Goulet, the director of the Milwaukee Yoga Center, designed and offers a weekly yoga class especially for people with PD. One can join exercise groups at a variety of venues as well.

Various walking aids including canes, walkers, transport chairs, and wheelchairs are available. I resisted each one because I was embarrassed. I worried I would be seen by a colleague or a student. Even with help, I am afraid I could trip in a restaurant or at a play. Peggy has urged me to ignore the stares and concentrate on what is working.

Involvement in groups that focus on leisure time activities, like reading, photography and gardening expands the lives of people with PD. After pushing myself, I have become more comfortable with being in public.

I am enjoying myself. The pain in my life has been balanced by the pleasure. Leaving the house, socializing, and expanding one's knowledge and skills are what matters. My efforts to discover and enjoy the positive in life are a victory—a mental and emotional transcendence over Parkinson's disease.

REFERENCES

Hyde, Trevor, Ph.D., personal conversation, September, 2011

Impact, AARP, January and February, 2006

Leo, Gary, D.O., "Attitude," *The Network*, Winter, 2011

Mamerow, Paul, P.A.-C., personal conversation, 2011

Marty, Diane, "Getting On Our Nerves," *E/The Environmental Magazine*, January 18, 2002

Nausieda, Paul, M.D., and Gloria Bock, *Parkinson's Disease: What You and Your Family Should Know*, National Parkinson Foundation, 2000

Parkinson's Action Network, "Hard Facts," May, 2002

Parkinson 's Disease Foundation, "Statistics on Parkinson's," and "Hope Through Research, Education, and Advocacy," Accessed October 3, 2011 http://www.pdf.org/en/parkinson statistics.s

Planet Ark, "Home Bug Spray May Increase Parkinson's Risk," study, May 8, 2000

Tönnies, Ferdinand, *Wikipedia, the Free Encyclopedia* vol. 102, p. 173-238

Walker, Jerry Jeff, Lines from his song . . . spoken by Paul Mamerow, P.A.-C. in a personal conversation, 2011

BIBLIOGRAPHY

Ahlskog, Eric J., *The Parkinson's Disease Treatment Book*, 2005

Argue, John, *Parkinson's Disease & The Art of Moving*, 2000

Blake-Krebs, Barbara, M.A. and Herman, Linda, MLS, *When Parkinson's Strikes Early*, 2001

Christensen, Jackie Hunt, *The First Year: Parkinson's Disease*, 2005

Fox, Michael J., *Lucky Man: A Memoir*, 2002

Graboys, Thomas, M.D., *Life in the Balance*, 2008

Havemann, Joel, *A Life Shaken: My Encounter with Parkinson's Disease*, 2002

Leo, Gary, D.O., *"Attitude", The Network*, Winter 2011

Lieberman, Abraham N., *Shaking up Parkinson's Disease: Fighting like a Tiger, Thinking like a Fox*, 2001

Lyons-Marjama, Jill, *What Your Doctor May Not Tell You About Parkinson's Disease*, 2003

Marty, Diane, *"Getting on Our Nerves," E/The Environmental Magazine*, 2002

Nausieda, Paul, M.D., and Gloria Bock, *Parkinson's Disease: What You and Your Family Should Know, National Parkinson Foundation*, 2000

Newsom, Hal, *HOPE: Four Keys to a Better Quality of Life for Parkinson's People*, 2006

Nutan, Sharma, M.D., *Parkinson's Disease and the Family: A New Guide*, 2005

Schwarz, Shelley Peterman, *Parkinson's Disease 300 Tips*, 2006

Walker, Jerry Jeff, *Ultimate Collection*, 2001

Weiner, William J., Shulman, Lisa M., Lang, Anthony E., *Parkinson's Disease: A Complete Guide for Patients and Families*, 2001

Wisniewski, Sandy Kamen, *I Can't Stop Shaking*, 2005

INDEX